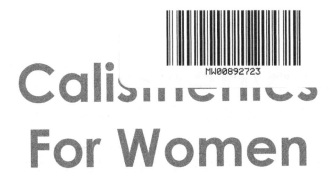

Calisthenics For Women

Female Body Workouts

Bodyweight Training and Movements

Dan C. Wilson

© 2015

Table of Contents

Introduction

Most muscle and strength books are dedicated to men. Aren't you tired of that? You keep hearing that women *shouldn't* work out, it will make them look bulky, muscles are for men, a girl with a six-pack is not attractive and the list goes on. I've decided to **dedicate** a book to <u>women</u>, because it's totally **possible** to have great power and be an *attractive* female.

In this book I will take you on a journey through the wonderful world of **calisthenics**. I can totally understand that you, as a female, don't want to look bulky and too muscled. Because frankly, most guys don't want their girlfriend to look stronger than them. You will find *great* exercises and tips in this book for ways to <u>improve</u> your strength and still keeping your **natural** female posture. I know that most weightlifting exercises can look a bit overwhelming and therefore, I believe that calisthenics is THE way to go for women!

My name is Dan C. Wilson and I've been involved and passionate about the sports and fitness industry for many years. Not only have I been a fitness instructor to numerous people, I have also completed many courses for being able to give you the best information and help you to overcome any health obstacle, which will sooner or later arrive in your life.

Calisthenics will make a *huge* difference in women's physically body, and will probably change your way of thinking forever. Get rid of the thoughts that working out with weights will make you look bulky, muscled and manly. It is one of the biggest *myths* in the fitness industry that I totally **disagree** with. In this book I want to share my thoughts and experience with you, and show you that calisthenics is absolutely <u>perfect</u> for women. Not only does it make you look great, it also burns fat way faster compared to working out on a treadmill. Lots of women went before you already, and they look stunning. Stop limiting your beliefs and *prove* others wrong!

This book will take you through the best calisthenics exercises, tips and benefits for **women**. Don't be afraid to grab some weights, because there <u>won't</u> be any weights. YOU are the weight. Calisthenics simply means *bodyweight training*, such as push-ups, sit-ups and pull-ups. Let's start today by slowly getting rid of the myths that women shouldn't work on their muscles.

Once you start getting results with the given bodyweight exercises in this book, you will finally understand that women <u>can</u> keep their female body shape while working out. Being a former gym instructor I can tell you that the secret for most muscled men is eating. That's right, **eating**. If you keep eating normal or less then you *won't* have to worry at all about gaining weight. Most people who want to become <u>bigger</u> and <u>stronger</u> start eating a lot, as the excessive foods will be converted to fats.

Now, that's normally not a very appealing method, BUT, fats will eventually be converted to more muscles as you work out. This feeds the growth of your body.

Another thing, women don't have the same **testosterone** level as men do. That means, even if you work out 5 times *harder* than they do, you will never achieve the same size without using supplements. Due to the testosterone difference, it's physically impossible. As this book is focused on calisthenics, you won't have to worry about not being able to achieve the same SIZE as males. Everybody should be able to perform the basic body exercises such as a push-up.

Let's get started and throw all the myths away about females not being able or shouldn't work on their muscles. Keep the intensity high and you won't get bigger. In case you're a woman that actually wants to become bigger and stronger than simply do the *opposite*.

Chapter 1:
Getting Started

This book is not about the concept and definition of calisthenics, so let's get started. But wait... **How** do we get started? Don't worry! The beauty of calisthenics is that you have absolute <u>freedom</u>. You don't need to buy fancy workout equipment or getting a gym subscription to get you started. Calisthenics is for **everyone, anywhere and anytime**.

That being said, absolute freedom doesn't *always* work out great for everyone. Especially if you're a beginner and you have no idea where to start or how to do things the **right** way. In general too much of anything is usually a bad thing, that can be the same with calisthenics. Too much freedom will result into confusion as there's no strict playground or time schedule. Especially if you're new to something, it's good to have a <u>guideline</u> that you can follow. In this book I'll hand you these guidelines so that you can get started and make adjustments as you become more experienced. We will build a **foundation** of strength and knowledge.

Let's not get too excited and overload our bodies with too many different exercises. We will start with the basics and slowly add more. If you've been neglecting sports for quite a while, don't fool yourself that you'll be able to start doing muscle-ups right off the bat after a year or two without any exercises.

First of all you need to make your body stronger by starting with the *basic* exercises. Getting familiar and stronger with the basic exercises such as push-ups, dips, pull-ups and squats is the most **important** part. All the more advanced exercises are a variation or combination of the basic exercises.

So getting the basics right will get you a long way.

In the 21st century, nowadays everybody is looking for shortcuts, secrets or magic supplements for reaching the goal faster and easier. Basically, we all like to do less and achieve **more**. The truth is, there are no healthy and natural shortcuts for your body. Although, I will share <u>FOUR</u> secrets with you about calisthenics, to build strength and keeping the right **female** shapes.

** 1. Be <u>patient</u>. Building your body into a better shape and gaining more power and strength takes time. Don't expect to turn into a superwoman overnight. Set **short term** and **small goals** to keep the *motivation* up, setting goals such as losing 30 kilogram is too significant and will be too far away. Cut your goals into smaller pieces, it shouldn't be a short term commitment but a <u>lifestyle</u>!

** **2**. Full body range motion. Doing things the incorrect way won't get you great results. It's very **important** to perform the exercises correctly. Always be aware of your body form and making the full range of motion. While performing your repetitions try to *control* your body throughout the whole exercise. It will make a HUGE difference in noticing results and success or simply wasting your time. Being able to perform 5 full motion range of push-ups is way better for your body to adapt in the **right** shape instead of doing 10 sloppy repetitions, just for the sake of the number. Become committed to a <u>clean form</u> and your body will shape and adapt itself to something **beautiful**.

** **3**. Female body shape. Don't add too **many** weight or extra repetitions. If you want your body to stay in shape, don't overdo your workout program. You want to make sure that you're keeping the intensity <u>high</u> so that your body will burn *fats*, but try avoiding adding too much weight on top of your own bodyweight. More repetitions, more sets and more weight will grow your body stronger faster but also bigger.

** **4**. Nutrition. Bodybuilders love consuming food. Consuming excessive food will make your body grow. Stick to a **diet** that's working for you and avoid eating too many *carbohydrates*. For a good fitness diet that supports your body, please refer to my ketogenic diet plan. You will find a preview at the end of this book or simply click the link below to get redirected to the ketogenic **4-week diet plan**.

Ketogenic Diet: Foolproof Diet Plan - Build a New Body in 4 Weeks With Quick & Fast Recipes (5 BONUS Recipes)

Keep those 4 secrets in mind and I can assure you that you will see great **results** without becoming too big and muscled!

Chapter 2:
Tips for Beginners

A common mistake of beginners is **incorrectly** performing the exercise. After spending many years in the gym myself as a fitness instructor, I've seen numerous people giving up as they *fail* to get results or due to neglecting keeping the <u>right body form</u>, ending up with *injuries* that prevents them from improving further.

As I gave out in the second tip on the previous page, it is very **important** perform the exercises *correctly*. It is way better to perform 5 accurate push-ups than doing 10 improper ones. If you're not doing the amounts you were hoping for, **never give up**! Success comes slow and steady. If you're able to do 5 pushups today, try to increase the amount to 6 during the next week. Little by little you will see *progress* and you'll get closer to your <u>goals</u>. Getting results takes time, so it's best to embrace that fact and be patient. Most people that you look up to have already been performing exercises for many years in a row.

If you feel that you've obtained a minor injury or a part of your body is becoming weaker, then <u>focus</u> on a different part of your body while giving your body enough time to fully **recover** the minor injury. In case your body is sensitive for injuries or you simply want to avoid them at all costs, then I'd highly suggest checking out my book about **stretching** exercises. By using the explained exercises as a warm-up and cooling down, you will *minimize* the chances and risks of getting injuries. I've left you a preview at the end of the book together with the diet plan, this additional information will surely <u>help</u> you even more to get the **best results** possible for you. If you're excited and you can't wait any longer, then look for the book title below to take you to the stretching book page.

<u>Stretching: Stretching Exercises for Beginners : Quick Ways to Become Flexible and Gain Strength</u>

Make calisthenics **fun** and discover the many exercises out there. Not only will you *reach* your goals, you'll also have more fun and you'll be able to stay *motivated* while achieving them. Note down your results, take note of your weight, write down the inches of your belly, do <u>everything</u> necessary to notice **improvements**. Sometimes it's hard for yourself to notice improvements when you look in the mirror every morning, however if you <u>write</u> the results down you'll be able to clearly see an increasing or decreasing number, depending on what your goals are.

If you want to **lose** some extra kilos next to gaining muscles and becoming stronger, start looking into *cardio* training. On top of that, follow the **ketogenic diet** that I've provided you! Take every little piece of information and absorb it. In case you want to gain additional weight, because you feel not comfortable with your current female body shape. Simply consume <u>more</u> food while you're having your breakfast, lunch and dinner. You might even want to take a look into *supplements* if you're not a big fan of eating. Supplements can help you immense to **gain** additional calories easily.

Lastly, make sure to get familiar with stretching exercises. This will help you to be more flexible and beneficial for muscle recovery. There's nothing more demotivating as obtaining an injury. You REALLY want to make sure that you're avoiding possible injuries while at the same time getting great flexibility, this will help you into forming a **perfect** body shape.

Chapter 3:
Beginners Workout Programs

If you're <u>not</u> a beginner, then feel free to skip this chapter. In case you're somewhat of a beginner, be it totally new or in the journey of your first weeks then I'd suggest to keep on reading. You don't want to miss out on **useful** information! I've given you an <u>easy-to-follow</u> program that is not too intense for beginners to execute, but will give you **great** results. I know it can be very difficult and hard to create a workout schedule, if you're new to something. So in this chapter I'll be handing out a beginner workout program to you. Feel free to swap exercises around to your likings, just make sure that you're aiming for the **same** muscle group if you choose to do so.

The amount of repetitions and sets is just an estimation, don't worry if you can't finish the beginner program. Stick to the exercises and <u>slowly</u> improve your numbers. There's no rush to achieve your goals! Slow and steady wins the race.

I have created <u>3</u> routines for you, which you can schedule in your week where you see fit. Don't *forget* to give your body enough rest to **recover**.

Beginner Routine #1:

<u>Pull-up</u> - Target: Biceps and Back
<u>Dips</u> - Target: Triceps
<u>Squats</u> - Target: Legs
<u>Inverted Rows</u> - Target: Chest

Try to complete 3 sets of each exercise, and 5 sets of squats. Aim for 10 repetitions per set, if your body is not able to perform the full 10 repetitions or the amount of sets, then stop just before you hit muscle failure – meaning that you've used up all your energy and strength in that part of your body. **Don't** force it, this may lead to injuries.

Not every beginner can *immediately* perform a full amount of pull-ups, as most are just not strong enough yet. Ask for assistance or perform negative pull-ups. The negative pull-up involves performing only the lowering phase of the exercise, and is a popular technique when building strength for full pull-ups. By performing the inverted rows, you can increase the difficulty of the exercise by positioning your body more horizontal.

Try to aim for 10 repetitions, if you decide to increase the difficulty. Don't increase weight or add resistance when you **cannot** reach 10 repetitions.

Beginner Routine #2:

Pull-up - Target: Biceps and Back
Dips - Target: Triceps
Squats - Target: Legs
Inverted Rows - Target: Chest
Split Squat – Target: Legs
Push-up – Target: Chest

The instructions for the second routine are the same as the first. Try to keep the intensity up, and do a full circle of every exercise with 1 set, and roughly **30 seconds** rest between every exercise. Try to aim for doing the full circle for 3 times.

Remember to always keep your body form **correct** and performing the exercises in <u>full range of motion</u>. Also don't forget to do **stretching** exercises before and after to minimize the risks of getting injuries.

Beginner Abdominals Routine:

Hanging Knee Raise – Target: Abs
1 Minute Elbow Plank – Target: Abs
Sit-up– Target: Abs

Try to complete every exercise with 3 sets, and work the list in a circle with **1 minute rest** between every 3 exercises. Aim for 10 repetitions while performing the hanging knee raises, and a maximum amount of sit-ups – as this is the last exercise before resting.

Calisthenics offers you a lot of different exercises to improve every part of your body separately that helps you to shape your body as a whole. When you become more experienced with different routines, exercises and training techniques, you'll be able to switch around exercises to create your **own** workout program and start becoming more comfortable with your own training sessions.

Now that you're more advanced, let's move on to the **3 best calisthenics workout programs** for more the more advanced athletes.

Chapter 4:
Calisthenics Exercises

You've become more advanced with calisthenics workout routines and you're now looking for different and **better** exercises to keep improving your results and creating variations of your current workout programs.

In this chapter I'll be handing out many of my <u>personal</u> best calisthenics exercises for you. All the exercises are based on bodyweight *without* the need of machines. We want to make sure everything is as **natural** as possible. These calisthenics exercises will give you the <u>best</u> improvement results to your strength and also physical level.

It can be difficult sometimes to improve your body *without* weights and machines, and surely it will ask a lot of your creativity to get into shape with a nice physique by only using your own bodyweight. That's why I'm here to help you. Plenty of exercises will be enough by just using your own bodyweight, should it be too light and easy – you can always ask someone around you to apply *slight* pressure and resistance to help <u>improve</u> your strength.

Starting from the next page, we'll examine the various exercises that you can implement in your workout routines. Note that *none* of the exercises are more significant than others, it's a personal creation that will improve **every** part of your body. Even though there will be favorites, make sure to routine the exercises, you want to work on every muscle of your body.

Let's take a look, shall we?

EXERCISES

Chest

Push-up

This is my all-time favorite calisthenics exercise to work on your upper body. Not only does it improve your chest, it also improves your triceps, pectorals and anterior deltoid. Make sure to keep the right body form, fully stretched and exercise in full motion range. Don't worry about adding weights before you can do at least a total of 25 push-ups in a row.

Incline Push-up

Same instructions as the normal push-up. Use a chair to perform the incline push-up. Make sure to keep your back straightened throughout the whole exercise.

Decline Push-up

The steepness level of the incline and decline push-up will make you focus more on different areas of your chest. Depending on the steepness you'll improve and work on your higher or lower part of the chest.

Incline Push-up

The incline is also a very powerful exercise to develop and strengthen your upper body. More specific, this will target more of the upper pectoralis compared to the regular push-up. To perform the incline push-up, simply start with the regular position but then elevate your feet on a bench or some other object.

Chest Dip

Another great exercise to improve and strengthen your upper body is the chest dip. Don't worry about not having the right equipment, you can simply put two chairs together for example. You'll have to be a little bit creative and make sure that whatever it is that you set up that it's safe and stable enough. Setting up a bad construction can lead to injuries, so again be careful how you set it up.

Back

Pull-up

By far the most powerful and favorite back exercise for great improvements. This exercise when done properly with full motion range will build a really beautiful shaped back. Try to find a safe and steady place to perform this exercise, in case you can't do the pull-ups yet then follow the instructions given in the beginner workout section.

Hyperextension

After the famous deadlift exercise, I believe this is one has earned a second place to strengthen the lower back. It can be a little bit tricky to find a good spot to do this, if you have not the right object to perform the hyperextension then simply ask someone to hold your feet so you don't fall. You'll be able to perform this exercise on the edge of a chair or bed for example. Make sure that the construction is steady, you don't want to fall over.

Underhand Pull-up

This is almost the same exercise as the regular pull-up, except you'll change your grip. The underhand grip allows you to lift more weight, so in case you weren't able to manage the regular pull-up, then you should have an easier time doing it with the underhand grip. It's also a great exercise to work on your biceps o top of your back.

Lying Torso Raise

A perfect exercise to work on your lower back and the upper glutes. Hold longer to intensify this exercise, for example 3-6 seconds.

Thighs

Squat

A very great exercise for females is squats. Not only will you work on making your thighs much stronger, you'll also work on your butt while doing it. You won't need any additional weight or construction to perform this exercise. Simply go down all the way deep and back up. In case the exercise is getting too light, and it takes too many repetitions to feel pressure then hold something heavy in your hands or ask someone to apply downward pressure to your shoulders. By far the best exercise to work on your quadriceps and butt.

Sissy Squat

A variation of the normal squat, and an excellent exercise for developing the quadriceps. A very important note during this exercise is to hold onto something while performing the exercise. Like the regular squat, if you need extra weight simply hold something heavy in one arm or ask someone else to put downward pressure to your shoulders.

Lunges

Another excellent exercise to develop the quadriceps. Make sure to do this exercise in full range of motion and get as low as possible. Should you feel that you need some resistance, then hold a random heavy object in your hands while going down. Keep focused on getting all the way down.

Split Single Leg Squat

This is almost the same as the regular squat exercise, except with the split single leg squat you'll have to place your leg up on a chair or a step for example and moving all the way down. Make sure that the construction is steady enough to support your weight while balancing your body.

Stiff-Leg Deadlift

It'll be slightly difficult to perform this exercise without additional weights, I'd suggest to hold a random heavy object in your hands should you need additional weight. If you don't have anything heavy around you, then ask someone to apply downward pressure to your shoulders. Always keep in mind to stay in the correct body form with a straightened lower back throughout the whole movement. If you don't add any weight or use any pressure or resistance, it will most likely only serve as a stretch. Another good way of adding resistance is to make someone sit down in front of you, when you're bending down at the lowest point, hold hands and make them press in the opposite direction as you go back up. Avoid any pulling, as this will make you lose your balance quite easily.

Calves

Calf Raise

An easy and yet powerful exercise. Stand on the edge of a step or any other sturdy object, and simply move down and stand on your toes as you go up. Holding a heavy object in your hands, or asking someone to put downward pressure to your shoulders will increase the difficulty. If you're close to a ceiling or something else, you can use your own arm strength as resistance by pushing down.

Seated Calf Raise

You'll be able to perform this exercise on any regular chair. However , you need a sturdy object in front of you where you can place your feet on. The great benefit about the calf raises are that you don't have to ask anyone or usually don't need any weights to intensify the exercise. On top of that you also train your arm strength while giving resistance to your quads.

Abdominals

Sit-up

Nothing fancy here, the regular sit-ups would do perfectly fine. Should you need additional weight in case the amount of repetitions are getting too high, simply hold something heavy in your hands and place it on your chest while performing the sit-ups. In case you don't have any heavy object near you, or you want to avoid using it. Then you can intensify the exercise by keeping your legs straight up in the air. The more you stretch your legs at 90 degrees, the more intense the exercise will become. Another way is to extend your arms above your head.

Lying Leg Raise

This exercise will focus on the lower abs. Lift up your torso to extend your legs upwards or hold legs slightly above the ground for a couple of seconds to intensify this exercise. Alternatively ask someone to push your legs down, avoid making your feet touch the ground for better results.

Twisting Crunches

The twisting crunches are a powerful way to increase your side abs. Lift up your legs like the normal sit-ups to intensify this exercise. Alternatively, if you get cramps in your legs – hold a heavy object in your hand and place it on your left or right chest as you move to the sides.

Chapter 5: Intermediate Workout Routines

Getting familiar with the different kind of exercises is always a good thing, but if you don't know *how* to put them in a good schedule, you'll be losing a lot of potential progress. It's very **important** to get as much variety in your calisthenics workout as you can while you're creating a workout routine. In case you're dealing with a busy schedule and want to do the minimum possible and still get some results, then I'd suggest sticking to <u>push-ups, squats and dips</u>. These 3 exercises are the most basic ones and will pretty much train your whole body without too much experience needed, compared to pull-ups for example.

However, should you want to get the <u>most</u> out of your workout, then it's necessary to dive deeper into the exercises and different kinds of variation so that you literally train every single muscle in your body. I've set up 2 routine programs that you can implement in your daily schedule.

They are based on **3 days** and **4 days** per week, in case you'd like to work out more then simply do a quick round of every muscle group, if you'd like to work out less per week then combine the days together.

The days are split up and focusing on 1 big muscle group together with a smaller one per day, and giving you an extra day of *rest* between your workouts. You could also choose to focus 3 days of your week on improving your muscles, and on the alternating days doing cardio for roughly 30 minutes.

Due to the nature of bodyweight exercises, I believe it is unnecessary to put an amount of repetitions to aim for. Simply try to reach for the **maximum** amount possible and move on to the next exercise.

THE 3-DAY ROUTINE

<u>Monday</u>
Target: Chest, Triceps and Abs
(2 sets, max reps) Push-up
(3 sets, max reps) Chest Dip
(2 sets, max reps) Decline/Incline Push-up
(3 sets, max reps) Sit-up

<u>Tuesday (OPTIONAL)</u>
30 Minutes cardio or light sets of strength exercises

<u>Wednesday</u>
Target: Back, Biceps and Abs
(2 sets, max reps) Pull-up
(3 sets, max reps) Hyperextension
(3 sets, max reps) Lying Torso Raise
(3 sets, max reps) Sit-up

<u>Thursday (OPTIONAL)</u>
30 Minutes cardio or light sets of strength exercises

<u>Friday</u>
Target: Thighs, Legs and Abs
(3 sets, max reps) Calf Raise
(2 sets, max reps) Stiff Leg Squat
(3 sets, max reps) Lunges
(2 sets, max reps) Squat

<u>Saturday</u>
Rest day

<u>Sunday</u>
Rest day

THE 4-DAY ROUTINE

Monday
Target: Legs
(3 sets, max reps) Squat
(2 sets, max reps) Lunges
(2 sets, max reps) Side Lunges
(3 sets, max reps) Step Up
(2 sets, max reps) Calf Raise
(2 sets, max reps) Stiff Leg Squat
(3 sets, max reps) Seated Calf Raise

Tuesday
Target: Back and Triceps
(2 sets wide grip, 1 set medium grip, max reps) Pull-up
(2 sets, max reps) Hyperextension
(3 sets, max reps) Lying Torso Raise
(2 sets, max reps) Decline Close Grip Push-up
(3 sets, max reps) Bench Dips

Wednesday (OPTIONAL)
30 Minutes cardio, light sets of strength exercises or extra abdominals day.

Thursday
Target: Chest and Biceps

(3 sets, max reps) Push-up
(2 sets of both, max reps) Incline/Decline Push-up
(3 sets, max reps) Chest Dip
(4 sets, max reps) Pull-up

Friday
Target: Abdominals

(3 sets, max reps) Sit up
(3 sets, max reps) Lying Leg Raise
(3 sets, max reps) Twisting Crunches

Saturday
Rest day

Sunday
Rest day

Chapter 6:
Female Butt Workout

We have finally made it to the **butt workout**! Having a toned and rounder butt is likely at the *top* of your calisthenics list, I have not forgotten about you! You're in the right place. In this chapter we will go through exercises that'll make your toned butt push your jeans to the absolute limit! Don't worry about going into the gym's weight room, after all this is still part of the calisthenics book.

After having completed the previous exercises and perhaps workouts, it's very tempting and easy to run back to the couch and start watching that lovely TV show. If you'd like to get a *bigger* and <u>rounder</u> butt, we're not quite done yet. This butt workout will make you obtain effective results in a **short** period of time. However, achieving your body shape goals ALWAYS has to be combined with the right **nutrition** plan. Follow the <u>Ketogenic Diet Plan</u> at the end of this book for a perfect sports diet that supports your body!

I know it can be very difficult staying *motivated* and going for the extra mile. Therefore, I've come up with **6 EASY butt exercises** that anyone can do at anytime and anywhere.

You won't even need to get out of the door or more specifically, leave your couch. These exercises are <u>easily</u> combined while watching TV or any other "lazy" activity. You'll be able to relax and without too much effort getting your butt in **perfect shape**.

I'm aware that men find it very important to have massive arms, or a big chest. This may possibly be as much important for women to have a big rounded butt. Don't be fooled by people who tell you that squats are the ONLY exercise that will make your butt rounder, bigger and firmer. There are **many** other exercises out there with different movements that will get you the same result.

In this chapter we'll be going through 6 butt exercises. If you're willing to do the work, you'll get the butt you were always dreaming of faster than you thought was possible.

Before we get started, I'd like you to go through **5 quick tips**:

** You won't be able to create a **round** butt by simply doing *light* exercises, use extra weights or resistance bands when possible. A round butt exists of muscles AND low body fat, therefore it's not only important to watch your nutrition closely but also you'd have to work on your **muscles**. If you follow the exercises explained in the previous chapters, you'll create a good basis of muscles for your butt.

** Forming a toned and round butt *without* gaining additional leg muscles is very hard and almost impossible. I've done my best to hand out 6 butt exercises that are mainly focused on building a round butt without overly simulating the leg muscles. Note that even though the primary and main focus is on the butt muscles, you'll most likely still slightly work on your leg muscles as well.

** The butt building process will require weights or resistance in order to obtain **fast** results. I want to avoid putting pressure on you, and you should be able to work on your butt by your own preferred speed. However, when you feel ready or it's taking you too long – add additional weights or use resistance bands for faster results.

** As with every physical activity, it's important to do a <u>proper</u> warm-up before you start working out to minimize risks to obtain injuries. It can easily happen that you get cramps in your leg or butt if you neglect a warm-up. Start the butt exercises light or without any weights at all, this will allow to increase the blood flow into your muscles.

** Again, use **full range motions** while performing the exercises. This is one of the most <u>important</u> things when you want to change your body shape. Doing the exercises improperly will not only cause injuries, but it will also not give you the preferred results either. **Slow and steady**! Keep the right body form in mind at all times.

Now that you're aware of the 5 tips, let's get started with the butt workout!

Donkey Kicks

- Place your body on your hands and knees, make sure to keep your core right and your back flat.
- Lift your right/left leg off the floor until your knee is in line with your hip, at roughly 90 degrees.
- We won't be pushing the leg as high as we can with this exercise, instead flex your foot and squeeze your glutes, this will make your heel raise slightly an inch towards the ceiling.
- Repeat this for 25 repetitions.
- Next up, move the knee that is in the air outside, make sure to keep your foot flexed and pulse your leg a small inch to the other side.
- Don't lift your leg up, just try to keep it at the same level.
- Do this for another 25 repelitions.

Glute Bridges

This exercise can be done in two different variations, both 25 repetitions.

1.
- Lie down on your back with your knees bent and keep your feet flat on the floor.
- (Optional) Place additional weight on your pelvic area.
- Make sure to keep your core tight, and raise your hips off the floor.
- Thrust them as high into the air as you can, while squeezing your glutes at the top.
- Don't move your shoulders off the ground.
- When lowering your hips back down, don't make your butt touch the floor before you go up again.

2.

- Sit down on your butt and place both hands behind you, pointing away from your body. Place roughly 12 inches away from you.
- Place your feet in front of you the same way as your hands.
- Squeeze your glutes as you move your butt upwards, creating a tabletop position.

Marching Bridge

- Lie down on your back with your hands placed next to your sides.
- Place your feet both on the ground and about 12 inches away from your pelvis.
- Push your body into a bridge position by using your heels, keep your spine straightened.
- Raise one leg and keep the other knee bent.
- Keep raising the leg until your hip is at 90 degrees.
- As you move your leg down, squeeze your glutes, this will prevent your pelvis falling down on the floor as you lower down your leg.
- Switch legs, and raise both legs 20 times.

Swimming Pilates

- Lie down on your stomach and stretch your arms fully in front of you, reaching overhead.
- Stretch out your legs to the other side and lift your arms, legs and head upwards.
- Keep your whole body straight during the full exercise.
- Lift 1 leg higher upwards together with the opposite arm.
- Once you lower them down, do the same for the other leg and arm.
- Keep your torso stable, and alternate sides in a slow and controlled manner.
- Raise both sides 20 times.

Side Saddle Leg Lifts

- Start on one side with both legs extended.
- Bend your leg that's supporting your body.
- Slide the leg in a 90 degree angle of your hip, this acts for stability.
- Place the lower arm under your head as support, upper arm can be placed on your hip.
- Flex your upper foot and lift it up for about 7 inches from the floor.
- Slight pulses upward should be made here for 20 repetitions.
- Once the 20 reps are finished, proceed with 20 circling movements with the same foot.
- Reset and repeat with the other foot.

Clam Pilates

- Place your body on one side, with your knees and hips bent in about 45 degrees on top of each other.
- Place your feet in line of your butt.
- Slightly lift your bottom waist off the floor while keeping everything tight.
- Raise the upper knee of your body towards the ceiling, don't lift your foot. Rinse and repeat for 20 repetitions.

Summarize

There you go! These are the **calisthenics** exercises you need to practice for getting your female body into shape and creating a tone butt. Just follow these exercises and workout routines and I can <u>assure</u> you that you'll see improvements faster than you thought.

Before you're heading out and start on your new calisthenics workout, let's have a **quick** look at everything that we've discussed in this book.

#1 - Getting Started

Starting out slow and steady is the <u>best advice</u>. Remember that slow and steady wins the race. Don't try to *rush* your journey into getting results. Usually this will only lead to disappointments and delays your progress as you'll end up with injuries as your body is not used to intense workouts. You can perform calisthenics exercises **anywhere** and at **any time**, no fancy machines are needed. Remember the <u>4 tips </u>and you'll see results soon enough!

#2 – Tips for Beginners

As explained in the first chapter, it's very important to watch your **nutrition**, you want food to support you rather than working against you. To *avoid* injuries, make sure to do the right and proper warming up together with a cooling down. Refer to my <u>stretching</u> book for the **best** exercises to minimize the risk of getting injuries. Perform your exercises with <u>full range of motion</u>, don't try to *rush* through it.

#3 – Beginners Workout Programs

3 Beginner workouts were handed out to you, stick to the workout routine and *slowly* improve your numbers. Don't worry too much about completing or improving the numbers yet, the beginner program is created to get you familiar with a variation of different calisthenics routines. Get familiar with them and then *slowly* move towards the intermediate workout programs. <u>Never give up</u>!

#4 – Calisthenics Exercises

You became more familiar with the different calisthenics exercises, as numerous exercises were handed out to you for working on every single part of your body. Note that *none* of the exercises are more significant than others, even though there are personal favorites, you'd want to experience and get familiar with every single one of the exercises. This will enable you to create your **own** workout routine in a later stage.

#5 – Intermediate Workout Routines

Getting familiar with the different kind of exercises is always a good thing, but if you don't know *how* to put them in a good schedule, you'll be losing a lot of potential progress. This is why I created 2 different intermediate workout routines for you. As you're becoming more and more advanced in the calisthenics world, I've created a **3-day** and a **4-day** workout program for you. Feel free to swap exercises around, but make sure that they are targeting the same muscle part of your body should you choose to do so. The workout programs are focusing on 1 big muscle group and 1 smaller one, keep this rule of thumb in mind whenever you're about to create your own routine.

#6 – Butt Workout

In this chapter we went through exercises that'll make your toned butt push your jeans to the absolute limit! These **6 butt exercises** will get you the butt you were always dreaming of faster than you thought was possible. If you're willing to do the work, of course. Next to 6 of the best butt exercises, I've given you **5 handful tips** to get the <u>best</u> results possible.

This book will guide you from a _beginner_ towards an **intermediate** calisthenics athlete with an _easy-to-manage_ process. Take it one step at a time and it won't be long until you're getting results and creating the body that you've always dreamed of.

All you have to do is take _action_.

You'll still need to work for it, but you can make it **easier** for yourself. Getting a _perfect female body_ shape doesn't always have to be a struggle and painful. Following my workout routines, exercises and tips should get you way ahead of the rest.

I hope you have found some of the answers you were looking for, and you're absolutely ready getting to the next level. All the information I've provided are through own experience and thorough research. You now have my best recommendations and advice that should get you a lot closer to your body shape goals.

Finally, if you enjoyed reading this book or have any feedback suggestions, then I would kindly ask you to leave a <u>review</u> behind on **Amazon**. Should you have suggestions for a subject in the future which you want to explore further, please let me know through the review button as well. It would be greatly appreciated by the community!

Thank you very much and I wish you all the luck towards your next goal.

Dan C. Wilson

About the author

It has been my passion and hobby to increase vitality and how to become the strongest and best version of yourself since 2009. The goals of my books are simple, it is to share powerful ideas that help us all to become stronger, healthier, more flexible in every way possible. Building strength and becoming the strongest version of yourself goes far beyond lifting heavy weights and growing muscle.

My books are all about having more vitality, flexibility, health, building better relationships, creating an attractive body, nutrition and abundance. In case you want to reach your full human potential on both mentally and physically aspect and become a strong and healthy looking person, who feels amazing every day and is respected and admired by friends, family and strangers, then you are definitely in the right place here.

It is my goal to help as many people as possible. That having said, in case I can change the life of one person and make that one person feel better and more successful in life, I have reached my goal. We are all in this together! You, me and everyone else in our community. Together we will work hard and spread the message of changing lives and make our surroundings stronger and healthier. We will create a healthier and stronger world!

Dan C. Wilson

Other books by Dan C. Wilson

Stretching: Stretching Exercises for Beginners –
Quick Ways to Become Flexible and Gain
Strength
By Dan C. Wilson (Author)

Find the benefits of stretching here! Proven
programs and exercises to improve muscle
flexibility and to avoid or recover injuries

You feel there is more to achieve with your
body, but you don't know where to start.
Everybody around you in the gym is making
steps forward, except you. Every day when
you look in the mirror you cannot see any
results. How come no matter how hard you
try, there is no progress at all?

This book will give you all the information you
need to accomplish the maximum flexibility
permitted by your body. You will learn the
importance of understanding the benefits of
stretching and why we should use them more
often in our daily life.

All the information provided to you in this book are through own experience as well as a high amount of research on the stretching topic to being able to only give you the best recommendations and suggestions out there. With the information of this book, you should be able to accomplish your maximum flexibility and strength permitted by your body structure.

Take action today and make the first step towards your success by downloading this book "Stretching Exercises for Beginners – Quick Ways to Become Flexible and Gain Strength".

Preview of "Stretching: Stretching Exercises for Beginners – Quick Ways to Become Flexible and Gain Strength".

Chapter 1:
Benefits of Stretching

Before we get straight down to the exercises, it is important to understand the benefits of stretching and why we should use them more often in our daily life. Any movement you make that requires moving a body part to the point at which there is an increase in the movement of a joint can be called a stretching exercise. There are many benefits gained from using a regular stretching program. I have listed down below some of the benefits of stretching for you.

- ✓ Good muscular and joint mobility.
- ✓ Improved appearance and self-image.
- ✓ Reduced injuries and pains – Use light stretches if the pain prevails.
- ✓ Improved muscular strength, flexibility and stamina – The benefit depends on the degree of how much stress you put on your muscle. For gaining more

*strength, medium or heavy stretches
are recommended. Further in this book
we will examine light, medium and
heavy stretching.*
- ✓ *Improved body alignment and posture.*
- ✓ *Prevention of back problems.*

*Good flexibility is known to bring positive
benefits in the muscles and joints. It aids with
injury prevention and helps you to minimize
muscle pains. Efficiency in all physical
activities will be improved and increasing
flexibility will also improve quality of life as well
as functional independence. Good flexibility
improves the elasticity of your muscles and
provides a wider range of motion in the joints.
Ease in body movements will be provided for
your everyday activities. A simple daily task
such as bending over and tying shoes is
accomplished better with flexibility.*

For every person, whether you are an athlete or not, a regular basic stretching program can bring some great benefits to you. Recent research studies on various injuries have shown that people with low flexibility have a highly increased chance of muscle injuries. However, the type of flexibility needed for reducing those injuries did not come from doing stretching exercises right before the activity as a warm-up. The flexibility required for a lower chance of getting injuries came from following a stretch training for a certain amount of weeks. Increased strength and endurance gains have been reported as well as improved flexibility and mobility.

A few general tips for when you are about to do your stretching exercises, try to include all the major muscle groups in your program. It is highly recommended to do at least two different stretches for each joint movement. In case you are about to start with a physical activity, use light stretches as part of your warm-up.

Once you are done with your exercise routine, cool down with light- or medium-intensity stretches. Should your muscles be sore after your exercises, try to use only light stretches ranging from two to three times. Should your muscle soreness or injury persist for several days, then I recommend to continue using light stretches only. It is very important to give your muscles enough rest to recover, instead of forcing it.

1.1
Know your Limits

Now that we know the many great benefits that stretching has to offer, it is also important to know your limits and what to avoid. Firstly, we will focus on the first step of any workout program. Knowing your limits. A workout should be something that you enjoy and look forward to, it should be a pleasurable part of your day. It can be the first thing you do in the morning when you wake up, or in the evening when you finished your working shift. There may be times you experience some muscle soreness while working out or after a workout, however, it should not be the type of pain that interferes with your functional behavior. The same theory goes for stretching. Stretching properly before, during and after a workout session, you will definitely decrease the chances of obtaining some serious injuries and you will avoid muscle soreness and pains.

It is therefore extremely important to know your body limits. Stretching is an activity that should improve your body stamina, rather than causing you pain. Stretching was invented to avoid pain and become more flexible. It might happen that you feel a small mild tension when you stretch, do not worry as this is just a temporary feeling from your body stiffness. In case you do feel any pain beyond the stiffness, you have gone too far and you should lower the tense level of your stretching.

Should you feel pain during stretching, this means that your body has employed its defense mechanism – the stretch reflex. This happens when you stretch your muscles and tendons to the point of pain. Your body has a safety measure to prevent some serious damage caused to the muscles and tendons. The stretch reflex is a protection of your muscles and tendons and prevents them from being stretched beyond their possible limits. Do never try to force your body beyond this protection point. You will risk causing serious damage to your muscle tissues, tendons and ligaments.

Ketogenic Diet: Foolproof Diet Plan - Build a New Body in 4 Weeks With Quick & Fast Recipes (5 BONUS Recipes)
by Dan C. Wilson (Author)

This book will give you all the information needed to accomplish the maximum results in weight loss with easy and quick recipes. You will be guided through a 4 week foolproof diet plan. You start exploring new benefits and you receive the best proven tips to stick to your diet plan to increase massive health benefits. The most effective recipes are handed to you in this book, with detailed information and specific amounts of calories, carbohydrates, fats, and proteins per meal. Your fridge and freezer have never looked so delicious before!

All the information provided in this book is through own experience as well as a high amount of research on the ketogenic topic to being able to only give you the best recommendations and suggestions out there. With the information of this book, you should be able to accomplish rapid weight loss and achieve great health results.

In this book you will read...

... Detailed information on Ketosis
... Benefits of Ketogenic
... THE Foolproof Diet Plan
... Delicious Daily Recipes
... Learning How to Create Your Own Diet Plan
... 5 BONUS Keto Recipes

Preview of "<u>Ketogenic Diet: Foolproof Diet Plan - Build a New Body in 4 Weeks With Quick & Fast Recipes (5 BONUS Recipes)</u>"

Chapter 1: Explanation of Ketogenic

In case you have read my CrossFit book, then you would have probably found a part of this information at the end of the book as a small bonus chapter and introduction to the ketogenic subject. I am aware that not everyone has read the CrossFit book yet, or is less interested in doing so compared to ketogenic diets. To make sure everyone is on the same level, I will bring it up for those who have missed it.

I can understand that not everyone is familiar with ketogenic diets, as I first heard about it roughly 3 years ago as well. Just like you, I was curious and eager to try it out. So far I have had really fantastic results, and I honestly believe in the validity of this diet. Both in terms of fat-loss, as in health-gain.

As ketogenic has been brought up not so long ago in this world, there is a lot of misconceptions about ketogenic diets and ketosis, I will try to summarize it in this chapter as detailed as possible, while at the same time trying to keep it short. I have provided a small 3-day introduction diet plan during the previous bonus, which I have left out in this book, since we will be going way more in depth in this ketogenic diet book, I will provide you many useful recipes together with a great diet plan that is easy to follow. In case you feel left out, I have given you a different kind of bonus at the end of this book, which I believe is a lot more helpful after going through the ketogenic diet plan!

Should you still be interested in the 3-day introduction ketogenic diet plan, then please follow the link below. You will find the content together with the introduction plan at the end of the CrossFit book. For the Kindle Unlimited users out there, it's free of charge and you can skip right to the end!

<u>CrossFit: Training Guide for Beginners - Become Stronger Today - Proven Programs, Exercises and Diets</u>

For everyone who is not familiar with ketogenic diets, you may be surprised how many benefits you will notice while following this very healthy diet.

A low-carb diet is often mistaken with a ketogenic diet, or the other way around. An important factor in whether or not a diet is ketogenic is the amount of carbohydrate. Simply stated; Ketosis means that the body is in a state where it lacks the availability of glucose to use as energy for your body. When that happens, your body will use a plan B, which is generating molecules called ketones instead of using glucose. Very interesting is that they serve the same use to equally energize our body. However, ketones have the ability to also provide most energy needed in the brain, where fatty acids cannot be used. Besides trying to force your body into a ketosis state to use ketone molecules, there is a fair amount of body tissues that prefer using ketones over glucose, for example your heart muscle.

A ketogenic diet is very well-known for being a low-carb diet. There are many different diets who all share the same focus, which is resulting the body of producing ketones in the liver to be used as energy. However, as the main focus may be the same, the standards are slightly different in every diet. In this book we will stick to the ketogenic standards.

The easiest molecule created to use as energy for your body is glucose. Food which contains a high amount of carbs will make your body produce glucose and insulin. This is the main reason why there are so many different diet plans out there with the main focus, which is basically avoiding high carbs foods. Glucose is easily produced by your body for energy, so your body will choose this molecule over any other energy source when it can. When your body has produced an amount of glucose, the insulin is produced to process the glucose in your bloodstream by channeling it around in the body.

Now that you have a bit more understanding on how the ketogenic diet works, you may realize now that as your body uses glucose as a primary energy source, your fats are not needed anymore and they will be stored. As you move on, and keep stacking on high-carb foods, your body will use the glucose again and again, and store the fats on top of the previous ones. When you choose to lower the intake of carbs, you will force the body into a state known as ketosis. Your body does not have glucose available, but it has to produce energy regardless of glucose. Your body will therefore start searching for alternative sources. This is the ketone molecule, the main focus of the ketogenic diet.

CPSIA information can be obtained at www.ICGtesting.com
Printed in the USA
BVOW06s0142121016

464810BV00008B/66/P